Living With Alzheimer's

Strategies for Patients and Caregivers

Rossana Lewis

TABLE OF CONTENT

Chapter 1: Understanding Alzheimer's Disease

1.1 What is Alzheimer's Disease?

1.2 Causes and Risk Factors

1.3 Diagnosis and Staging

Part I: Coping with Alzheimer's as a Patient

Chapter 2: The Alzheimer's Journey

2.1 Early Symptoms and Challenges

2.2 Navigating the Middle Stages

2.3 Late-Stage Alzheimer's and End-of-Life Considerations

Chapter 3: Building a Support System

3.1 The Role of Family and Friends

3.2 Joining Support Groups

3.3 Working with Healthcare Professionals

Chapter 4: Cognitive and Emotional Wellbeing

4.1 Maintaining Cognitive Function

4.2 Managing Anxiety and Depression

4.3 Coping with Memory Loss

Part II: Providing Care as a Caregiver

Chapter 5: Understanding Caregiving
5.1 The Caregiver's Role and Challenges
5.2 Legal and Financial Considerations
5.3 Balancing Caregiving with Personal Life

Chapter 6: Effective Communication
6.1 Communicating with a Loved One with Alzheimer's
6.2 Dealing with Challenging Behaviors

Chapter 7: Creating a Safe and Supportive Environment
7.1 Home Safety Tips
7.2 Daily Routine and Structure
7.3 Managing Medications and Appointments

Chapter 8: Self-Care for Caregivers
8.1 Recognizing Burnout and Compassion Fatigue
8.2 Strategies for Self-Care

8.3 Respite Care and Seeking Help

Part III: Strategies and Resources

Chapter 9: Lifestyle and Alzheimer's
9.1 Nutrition and Diet
9.2 Exercise and Physical Activity
9.3 Cognitive Stimulation

Chapter 10: Promising Therapies and Research
10.1 Current Treatment Options
10.2 Emerging Therapies and Clinical Trials
10.3 The Search for a Cure

Chapter 1: Understanding Alzheimer's Disease

1.1 What is Alzheimer's Disease?

Alzheimer's disease is the most common type of dementia. It is a progressive disease beginning with mild memory loss and possibly leading to loss of the ability to carry on a conversation and respond to the environment. It involves parts of the brain that control thought, memory, and language. It can seriously affect a person's ability to carry out daily activities. The number of people living with the disease doubles every 5 years beyond age 65.

This number is projected to nearly triple to 14 million people by 2060.1

Symptoms of the disease can first appear after age 60, and the risk increases with age. Younger people may get Alzheimer's disease, but it is less common.

1.2 Causes and Risk Factors

There are many different things that can increase a person's chances of getting Alzheimer's. These are known as 'risk factors'. Some of these risk factors cannot be changed, but many others can.

Risk factors that cannot be changed includes:

Age: Age is the biggest risk factor for Alzheimer's, as it is for most types of dementia. This means that a person is more likely to get Alzheimer's as they get older. Above the age of 65, a person's risk of developing Alzheimer's doubles about every five years.

Although most people with Alzheimer's are over 65, younger people can also get it. Around one in three people with young-onset dementia have Alzheimer's.

Sex: There are about twice as many women over 65 with Alzheimer's as there are men over 65 with the condition. This is mostly because women tend to live longer than men.

However, women over the age of 80 still have a slightly higher risk of getting Alzheimer's than men their age. We don't know the exact reasons for this.

There has been a lot of interest in how menopause may increase a person's risk of getting Alzheimer's. While it seems that very early menopause caused by medical treatment can increase risk, it's still unclear if it's also a risk factor when it happens more naturally.

Genes

There are certain genes that may be passed down (inherited) from a parent that can affect a person's chances of getting Alzheimer's. There are two types of these genes: 'familial' genes and 'risk' genes.

Familial genes will definitely cause Alzheimer's if they are passed down from a parent to a child. Out of 1000 people who have Alzheimer's, less than ten of those people will have it because of a familial gene.

Risk genes increase a person's chances of developing Alzheimer's. They are much more common than familial genes. However, unlike familial genes, risk genes do not always cause a person to develop the condition. Most of them only slightly increase a person's risk.

People with Down's syndrome have a much higher risk of developing Alzheimer's disease because of a difference in their genes.

Risk factors that can be controlled:

Lifestyle: People who live a healthy lifestyle, especially from mid-life (age 40–65) onwards, are less likely to develop Alzheimer's. This includes not smoking, not drinking too much alcohol, and eating a healthy balanced diet.

Keeping physically, mentally and socially active may help a person to reduce their risk of developing Alzheimer's.

Protecting the head from injuries throughout a person's life may potentially reduce the risk of Alzheimer's. Traumatic brain injuries (TBIs) are caused by a blow or jolt to the head, especially if the person is knocked out unconscious.

Health Conditions: There are lots of health conditions that increase a person's risk of developing Alzheimer's disease (as well as vascular dementia).

These includes:

- diabetes, stroke and heart problems
- risk factors for heart and blood vessel disease, such as high blood pressure, high cholesterol and obesity in mid-life
- age-related hearing loss
- depression.

Managing these conditions and getting support from health professionals as early as possible may help you to reduce your risk.

1.3 Diagnosis and Staging

An important part of diagnosing Alzheimer's disease includes being able to explain your symptoms. Input from a close family member or friend about your symptoms and their impact on your daily life helps. Tests of memory and thinking skills also help diagnose Alzheimer's disease.

Blood and imaging tests can rule out other potential causes of the symptoms. Or they may help your health care professional better identify the disease causing dementia symptoms.

In the past, Alzheimer's disease was diagnosed for certain only after death when looking at the brain with a microscope revealed plaques and tangles. Health care professionals and researchers are now able to diagnose

Alzheimer's disease during life with more certainty. Biomarkers can detect the presence of plaques and tangles. Biomarker tests include specific types of PET scans and tests that measure amyloid and tau proteins in the fluid part of blood and cerebrospinal fluid.

Diagnosing Alzheimer's disease would likely include the following tests:

Physical and Neurological Exam: A health care professional will perform a physical exam. A neurological exam may include testing:

- Reflexes.
- Muscle tone and strength.
- Ability to get up from a chair and walk across the room.
- Sense of sight and hearing.
- Coordination.

- Balance.

Lab Tests: Blood tests may help rule out other potential causes of memory loss and confusion, such as a thyroid disorder or vitamin levels that are too low. Blood tests also can measure levels of beta-amyloid protein and tau protein, but these tests aren't widely available and coverage may be limited.

Mental Status and Neuropsychological Testing: Your health care professional may give you a brief mental status test to assess memory and other thinking skills. Longer forms of this type of test may provide more details about mental function that can be compared with people of a similar age and education level. These tests can help establish a diagnosis and serve as a starting point to track symptoms in the future.

Brain Imaging: Images of the brain are typically used to pinpoint visible changes related to conditions other than Alzheimer's disease that may cause similar symptoms, such as strokes, trauma or tumors. New imaging techniques may help detect specific brain changes caused by Alzheimer's, but they're used mainly in major medical centers or in clinical trials.

Imaging of brain structures include:

- Magnetic resonance imaging (MRI). MRI uses radio waves and a strong magnetic field to produce detailed images of the brain. While they may show shrinkage of some brain regions associated with Alzheimer's disease, MRI scans also rule out other conditions. An MRI is generally preferred to a CT scan to evaluate Alzheimer's.

- Computerized tomography (CT). A CT scan, a specialized X-ray technology, produces cross-sectional images of your brain. It's usually used to rule out tumors, strokes and head injuries.

Future Diagnostic Tests: Researchers are working to develop tests that can measure biological signs of disease processes in the brain. These tests, including blood tests, may improve accuracy when making a diagnosis. They also may allow the disease to be diagnosed before symptoms begin. A blood test to measure beta-amyloid levels is currently available.

Genetic testing isn't recommended for most people being evaluated for Alzheimer's disease.

But people with a family history of early-onset Alzheimer's disease may consider it. Meet with a genetic counselor to discuss the risks and benefits before getting a genetic test.

Stages of Alzheimer's Disease

Alzheimer's disease typically progresses slowly in three stages: early, middle and late (sometimes referred to as mild, moderate and severe in a medical context). Since Alzheimer's affects people in different ways, each person may experience dementia symptoms or progress through the stages differently.

Early-stage Alzheimer's (mild): In the early stage of Alzheimer's, a person may function independently. He or she may still drive, work and be part of social activities. Despite this, the person may feel as if he or she is having memory lapses, such as forgetting familiar words or the location of everyday objects.

Middle-stage Alzheimer's (moderate): Middle-stage Alzheimer's is typically the longest stage and can last for many years. As the disease progresses, the person with Alzheimer's will require a greater level of care.

During the middle stage of Alzheimer's, the dementia symptoms are more pronounced. the person may confuse words, get frustrated or angry, and act in unexpected ways, such as refusing to bathe. Damage to nerve cells in the brain can also make it difficult for the person to express thoughts and perform routine tasks without assistance.

In the middle stage, the person living with Alzheimer's can still participate in daily activities with assistance. It's important to find out what the person can still do or find ways to simplify tasks. As the need for more intensive care increases, caregivers may want to consider respite care or an adult day center so they can have a temporary break from caregiving while the person living with Alzheimer's continues to receive care in a safe environment.

Late-stage Alzheimer's (severe): In the final stage of the disease, dementia symptoms are severe. Individuals lose the ability to respond to their environment, to carry on a conversation and, eventually, to control movement. They may still say words or phrases, but communicating pain becomes difficult. As memory and cognitive skills continue to worsen, significant personality changes may take place and individuals need extensive care.

The person living with Alzheimer's may not be able to initiate engagement as much during the late stage, but he or she can still benefit from interaction in ways that are appropriate, like listening to relaxing music or receiving reassurance through gentle touch. During this stage, caregivers may want to use support services, such as hospice care, which focus on providing comfort and dignity at the end of life. Hospice can be of great benefit to people in the final stages of Alzheimer's and other dementias and their families.

Part I: Coping with Alzheimer's as a Patient

Chapter 2: The Alzheimer's Journey

2.1 Early Symptoms and Challenges

Alzheimer's is a brain disease that causes a slow decline in memory, thinking and reasoning skills. There are 10 warning signs and symptoms. If you notice any of them, don't ignore them. Schedule an appointment with your doctor.

Memory Loss that Disrupts Daily Life: One of the most common signs of Alzheimer's disease, especially in the early stage, is forgetting recently learned information. Others include forgetting important dates or events, asking the same questions over and over, and increasingly needing to rely on memory aids (e.g., reminder notes or electronic devices) or family members for things they used to handle on their own.

Challenges in Planning or Solving Problems: Some people living with changes in their memory due to Alzheimer's or other dementia may experience changes in their ability to develop and follow a plan or work with numbers. They may have trouble following a familiar recipe or keeping track of monthly bills. They may have difficulty concentrating and take much longer to do things than they did before.

Difficulty Completing Familiar Tasks: People living with memory changes from Alzheimer's or other dementia often find it hard to complete daily tasks. Sometimes they may have trouble driving to a familiar location, organizing a grocery list or remembering the rules of a favorite game.

Confusion with Time or Place: People living with Alzheimer's or other dementia can lose track of dates, seasons and the passage of time. They may have trouble understanding something if it is not happening immediately. Sometimes they may forget where they are or how they got there.

Trouble Understanding Visual Images and Spatial Relationships: Some people living with Alzheimer's or other dementia could experience vision changes. This may lead to difficulty with balance or trouble reading. They may also have problems judging distance and determining color or contrast, causing issues with driving.

New Problems with Words in Speaking or Writing: People living with Alzheimer's or other dementia may have trouble following or joining a conversation. They may stop in the middle of a conversation and have no idea how to continue or they may repeat themselves. They may struggle with vocabulary, have trouble naming a familiar object or use the wrong name (e.g., calling a "watch" a "hand-clock").

Misplacing Things and Losing the Ability to Retrace Steps: A person living with Alzheimer's or other dementia may put things in unusual places. They may lose things and be unable to go back over their steps to find them again. He or she may accuse others of stealing, especially as the disease progresses.

Decreased or Poor Judgment: Individuals living with Alzheimer's or other dementia may experience changes in judgment or decision-making. For example, they may use poor judgment when dealing with money or pay less attention to grooming or keeping themselves clean.

Withdrawal from Work or Social Activities: A person living with Alzheimer's or other dementia may experience changes in the ability to hold or follow a conversation. As a result, they may withdraw from hobbies, social activities or other engagements. They may have trouble keeping up with a favorite team or activity.

Changes in Mood and Personality: Individuals living with Alzheimer's may experience mood and personality changes. They can become confused, suspicious, depressed, fearful or anxious. They may be easily upset at home, with friends or when out of their comfort zone.

2.2 Navigating the Middle Stages

For some patients, the middle stage is considered the most difficult. Your memory slowly start to fade and you may start to forget things like people's names or a home address. Or perhaps, you may feel angry trying to do a task which seem overwhelming. As this disease progresses, you may find yourself feeling helpless. Here are some tips on how to handle the moderate stage of this disease:

Gentle Reminders: In middle-stage Alzheimer's, damage occurs in the parts of the brain that controls reasoning, decision making, and sensory processes. You may likely experience more rapid memory loss and the ability to perform basic routines. One way to bypass this is through gentle reminders, you can set alarms on your phone with the description written out bold on what to do during that period. Use very specific phrases in description to understand clearly.

Help Calm Sundowning: Roughly 20% of Alzheimer's individuals experience increased agitation or restlessness at night. Referred to as "sundowning," these late-in-day behavioral problems can disturb the sleep cycle. Medical professionals haven't been able to explain the exact cause of sundowning but have come up with a few tips to help combat the problem. It is best to be very active during the day so at night you can get tired and sleep to avoid being restless. Encourage yourself to participate in more challenging activities such as going to a doctor's appointment or even bathing. We also suggest incorporating some simple exercises earlier in the day. When it is time for bed, make sure the room is at a comfortable temperature with the proper safety precautions in place such as night lights and window locks.

Create Meaningful Activities: Besides providing a relaxing feeling, activities can reduce wandering and agitation. "Meaningful activities" doesn't necessarily mean creating new things to do every day. It simply means doing something that will inspire self-confidence in you. You can prepare dishes, do arts and crafts or just go for a walk. No matter how simple the activity is, it can encourage you to express yourself through different means whether through art or an old hobby you use to love.

Build your Support System: You can ask for help as caring for yourself alone could be so exhausting. If you need to reach out for help, be very specific in what you need. And if someone feels reluctant to help, don't take it personally as dealing with Alzheimer's disease may be demanding.

2.3 Late Stage Alzheimer's and End-of-Life Considerations

People with Alzheimer's disease can have a good quality of life for some time. But at some point, medical care must focus on how to keep them comfortable. It's important to get ready for this time and make a plan before it comes. You should also know what services are available when you need them. These include medical professionals, hospice services, nursing homes, and assisted living.

There are end-of-life services including palliative (comfort) care designed to ease pain for anyone with a serious long term illness like Alzheimer's. Hospice care, which is only for people who feel they have 50% chances of not living more than 6 months. It's designed to make the process of dying as comfortable as possible. Both types of care can be given at home, in a nursing home, assisted living facility or in the hospital.

The best way to get ready for the final stages of your Alzheimer's disease is to know your wishes, get your will and other financial plan in order, decide where you want to be let at rest, find out about hospice, palliative care, and other services available in your area and what your insurance will cover.

The way people with Alzheimer's disease die is different from person to person, but there's a basic pattern to the process. They slowly lose the ability to control basic body functions, such as eating, drinking, and toileting. After a while, their body shuts down. They can't move much on their own. They don't want to eat or drink and they lose weight. They often get seriously dehydrated. It can get hard for them to cough up fluid from their chest.

It is very common for people with Alzheimer's to lose their appetite and not want to eat. You may think about using a feeding tube, but these tend to be uncomfortable. They also cause other physical problems, so they don't make people with this disease live longer. If you force yourself to take a fluid or drink, it may gather in your lungs and make it hard for you to breathe. This is why doctors don't recommend that tube be used for people with this disease.

It may also be difficult to communicate and your loved ones may not know when you're in pain. You can express your pains for them to understand through facial expressions, grunts and sighs. Talk to your doctor if you feel severe pains.

Chapter 3: Building a Support System

3.1 The Role of Family and Friends

Caring for a loved one with Alzheimer's is a profound and often challenging journey requiring more than just medical attention. It demands a comprehensive support system that encompasses emotional, practical, and social elements. Alzheimer's is a neurodegenerative condition that not only affects the individual diagnosed but also has a ripple effect on their loved ones. Building a robust support network that includes family, friends, and the broader community is crucial for providing sustainable and compassionate long-term care.

Family members are often the first line of support for individuals with Alzheimer's. Spouses, children, and siblings are faced with the challenge of not only understanding the disease but also adjusting their own lives to provide care, especially if it is long-term. Open communication within the family is vital to ensure everyone is on the same page regarding care decisions, treatment plans, and the emotional challenges that arise. Siblings can provide additional support by sharing responsibilities and allowing primary caregivers to take necessary breaks. Dividing tasks such as doctor appointments, meal preparation, and medication management can help distribute the load while maintaining a high standard of care.

One of the most challenging decisions families often face during Alzheimer's care is whether to move their loved one to a care facility. This decision is deeply emotional and complex, considering the individual's safety, well-being, and quality of life. Family unity becomes paramount during these moments. Open communication, understanding each member's perspectives and shared decision-making are crucial. While opinions may differ, it's important to remember that the ultimate goal is the best possible care for the individual with Alzheimer's. Working together, families can ensure that this decision is made with love, compassion, and the best interests of their loved ones at heart.

Friends play a unique role too in providing emotional support for caregivers and the individual with Alzheimer's. While they might not be directly involved in day-to-day caregiving tasks or providing long-term care, their presence can offer much-needed respite and a sense of normalcy. Spending time with friends who understand the situation and offer nonjudgmental companionship can help caregivers recharge and maintain their mental well-being. Friends can also engage in simple activities with the individual with Alzheimer's, such as taking walks, playing games, or sharing stories from the past. These interactions contribute to the person's social engagement and cognitive stimulation, both of which are crucial for maintaining a sense of self.

The role of the community is often underestimated in Alzheimer's care, but it can have a significant impact. Community resources, support groups and local organizations focused on Alzheimer's can provide caregivers with valuable information, advice, and a sense of belonging. Attending support groups allows caregivers to share their experiences, exchange coping strategies, and gain insights from others facing similar challenges. Community organizations can also provide practical help. These resources help caregivers build their skills, manage stress, and navigate the complex world of Alzheimer's care more effectively.

3.2 Joining Support Groups

Alzheimer's disease is a common form of dementia that can be challenging for those with the condition and the people who care for them. Support groups may help provide these individuals with emotional support and a sense of community. In-person and online Alzheimer's support groups are available across the United States. There are also groups for caregivers.

Although the specifics can vary between organizations, these groups may provide emotional and mental health support and resources about the condition.

In-person Alzheimer's support groups typically offer local meetings for people with the condition.

A person can search online for organizations that operate in their area. For example, the Alzheimer's Association has many regional chapters that offer local services for people living with Alzheimer's disease and their caregivers. Its website has a search tool to help people find their nearest chapter.

Though services may vary depending on location, some services they offer include:

- support for individuals with Alzheimer's and those who support people with the condition
- information and news about Alzheimer's disease
- volunteer opportunities
- fundraising events

People who have Alzheimer's or care for a person with the condition can also ask a doctor about local organizations offering in-person support groups. Alternatively, social workers at a hospital or other healthcare professionals may be able to help with finding them.

Online Alzheimer's support groups may provide similar benefits to in-person support groups, including:

- support for emotional needs and mental health
- help with answering questions and finding resources
- connecting with others
- fundraising opportunities
- events

An additional advantage may be the ease of access. People can often connect with people at their convenience online and join a group from anywhere. This may be particularly useful for people in rural areas who cannot find an in-person support group nearby.

3.3 Working with Health Care Professionals

Leaving the person living with Alzheimer's in the care of another is never an easy thing to do. But by working closely with providers and staying involved in care, you can help ensure all care needs of the person with Alzheimer's are being met.

First, you must prepare caregivers in the sense that you must familiarize them with the needs and history of yourself or the person living with Alzheimer's. Tell them the person's place of birth, childhood memories, family stories, favorite hobbies, occupation, likes, dislikes, and morning and evening routines.

Second, a care plan should be written that documents care and support needs of the person with Alzheimer's. An in-home care agency or care community will work with you to develop care plans for the person with Alzheimer's. You will provide insights about the person's preferences and routines. If possible, the person living with Alzheimer's should be involved in the care planning. As the disease progresses, the person's needs will change and, in some cases, a particular type of care may no longer be suitable. As this occurs, the care plan will also change. Ask the care provider how often care plans are reviewed and care conferences are held.

Third, there should be adequate communication. Schedule regular meetings or telephone calls with care providers. Discuss the care plan, any changing needs and concerns. Also give helpful feedback and praise good work

Chapter 4:Cognitive and Emotional Well-Being

4.1 Maintaining Cognitive Functions

Participating in stimulating cognitive activities can help improve memory, problem-solving skills, and language abilities.

Memory games are good examples which challenge the memory such as word games, crossword puzzles and memory matching games, which can help improve cognitive function and stimulate memory recall. These types of games can be adapted to the person's level of ability and can provide an enjoyable way to exercise the brain.

Second, Reminiscence therapy encourages people with Alzheimer's to recall and talk about past events and memories. This helps stimulate cognitive function and improves memory retrieval. Reminiscing about familiar topics or events from the past can also provide a sense of familiarity and comfort.

Third, reading can be an excellent cognitive stimulation activity, especially if the person has enjoyed reading in the past.
Reading books, magazines, or newspapers can help improve language skills, promote concentration, and engage the imagination.

4.2 Managing Anxiety and Depression

Anxiety and depression can be managed depending on the person's needs. If a person with Alzheimer's has mild anxiety, it may help to listen to their worries and reassure them. Many things can cause anxiety or make it worse. Addressing these as much as possible can help make a person feel less anxious. For example, if they are worried that they will lose their balance and fall, doing things to stop this from happening can help to make them feel less anxious. This could include encouraging the person to do exercises to become physically stronger, installing grab rails or reducing any clutter in their environment. It may help to adapt a person's home so it feels calmer, safer and less stressful.

If pain is contributing to the person's anxiety and depression, they should have regular pain relief to help them feel more comfortable. If they are worried about becoming lonely or cut off from people, their friends and family members can help to make them feel included and remain socially active. Reducing depression can involve a range of people. This can include the person's family and friends as well as professionals, such as GPs, psychotherapists, occupational therapists, physiotherapists and social workers.

People with more severe and persistent anxiety and depression may benefit from psychological therapies such as cognitive behavioral therapy (CBT). There is also evidence that doing music therapy (with a qualified therapist) reduces agitation. Some people may be prescribed medication to treat their anxiety.

4.3 Coping with Memory Loss

There are so many ways one can cope with memory loss especially if he/she is diagnosed with Alzheimer's. The following are tips to help you cope with memory loss:

Build on the Skills you Still Have: You will still have skills even if you have memory problems. For example, if you've always been an organizer and good at planning, make the most of this when facing new challenges.

Stay in a Regular Routine: Set up a regular daily routine. This will make it easier to remember what will happen over the course of the day. Include time to relax as part of the routine. Keep some variety and stimulation, such as meeting up with a friend or going out to the shops, so you don't get bored.

Try to Manage your Time: Don't be too hard on yourself if you find something more difficult than you used to. You could take some time out and come back to it again later, or think about different ways to manage the task. You could make a note to finish the task as a reminder to yourself later on. Try to do the most challenging things at the time of day when you have the most energy and can concentrate best. Avoid them if you feel tired, anxious, or unwell. Take your time.

Talk About Your Day: If you've been out for the day, talk to your partner, or a friend or family member afterwards about it. This is a good way of remembering and feeling positive about what you've done that day.

Plan Ahead: Plan ahead to make your daily tasks more manageable. For example, put the things you'll need for the next day near the front door.

You could put out your bag, your keys, and your wallet or purse. This will help you to remember to take these items with you.

Do One Thing at a Time: Try to do only one thing at a time. For example, if you're making a cup of tea, don't make a phone call at the same time. For a new task, repeat it and give yourself time to learn it.

Take Small Steps: Break tasks down into smaller steps. Then you can focus on just one step at a time. For example, if you're wet-shaving or washing your hair, set out the things you need in order then put each one aside once you've used it. Ask for help from others if you think you need it.

Keep One Place for Everything you Need: Try to keep important items such as your keys, glasses, purse or wallet in the same place. This could be a large bowl somewhere obvious and visible (for example, by the telephone, near the front door, or on the coffee table). Then you can always find them easily.

Simplify the Layout of Your Home: Try to keep the layout of your home familiar so that you know where things are. Consider labeling drawers and cupboards with words or pictures of what's inside them. Remove any clutter or unnecessary items.

Reduce Distractions: If your environment is noisy or very busy, you will find it harder to remember things or concentrate. Your memory works much better with no distractions. Try to make your environment quiet and remove any unnecessary distractions.

Get Support: Talk to friends and family about how you feel and how you can work together. They can support you to try out new techniques to help with your memory.

Part II: Understanding Care as a Caregiver

Chapter 5: Understanding Caregiving

5.1 The Caregiver's Role and Challenges

An Alzheimer's caregiver provides ongoing and quality care to patients of this disease. General responsibilities include discreet assistance with the activities of daily living, such as bathing, dressing and incontinence. Dementia caregivers also provide various types of additional in-home support. The following are the roles of a caregiver in respect to this context:

Medication Reminders: A physician may prescribe medications that can temporarily reduce it's symptoms. An Alzheimer's patient may have difficulties in remembering when and how to take the medications. It is your work as the caregiver to remind them, guide them so the take these medications judiciously.

Routines: Alzheimer's patient thrive with daily routines. Patterns in everyday life help them know what to expect and to continue achieving these things on their own. As a result, Alzheimer's patient who are guided by daily routines are more likely to feel confidence and dignity. Alzheimer's caregivers promote routines in everyday living. The professionals establish set times for meals, bathing and grooming. A patient who is used to bathing in the morning can continue doing so under the caregiver's care.

Wandering Prevention: Any patient who suffers from memory problems and is mobile is at risk for wandering. Disorientation and confusion are common symptoms even in the early stages of Alzheimer's. Wandering can be extremely dangerous, as patients may become lost or hurt. Alzheimer's caregivers help prevent a patient from wandering. Structured days can lower the chances of wandering. If wandering is likely to occur at specific times, the caregiver will plan activities to reduce restlessness. Caregivers offer reassuring words when the patient needs to go home.

Safety: Care recipient safety is a high priority for caregivers. A patient may turn on the stove and forget to turn it off. A watchful caregiver will prevent a kitchen fire. Caregivers provide continued supervision at home, while being careful to never leave the patient alone in a vehicle.

There are different challenges a caregiver faces while caring for an Alzheimer's patient.

Physical and Emotional Demands: Caregiving for an Alzheimer's patient can be physically and emotionally draining. The person with Alzheimer's requires constant attention and care, and the caregiver must be available at all times. This can lead to physical exhaustion and emotional stress. Alzheimer's patients may also have difficulty sleeping, which can disrupt the caregiver's sleep patterns as well. Caregiving is a full-time job that requires patience, compassion, and understanding.

Behavioral Changes: Alzheimer's disease is known for causing behavioral changes in patients. These changes can range from irritability and agitation to depression and anxiety. A caregiver must be prepared to handle these behavioral changes and know how to de-escalate any potentially dangerous situations. This can be incredibly challenging, as Alzheimer's patients may not respond to reason or logic.

Financial Strain: Alzheimer's disease can be expensive to manage. Medications, doctor visits, and other medical expenses can quickly add up. The caregiver may need to take time off work or reduce their work hours to care for the patient, which can lead to a loss of income. This financial strain can be overwhelming for caregivers, especially if they are already struggling to make ends meet.

Social Isolation: Caregiving for an Alzheimer's patient can be isolating. The caregiver may not have time to socialize with friends or participate in activities they enjoy. They may also feel uncomfortable leaving the patient or loved one alone or with someone else. This can lead to feelings of loneliness and depression, which can further impact their mental health.

Caregiver Burnout: Caregiving for an Alzheimer's patient can be emotionally draining, and caregivers may experience burnout. Burnout is a state of physical, emotional, and mental exhaustion that can occur when caregivers don't take care of themselves. This can lead to feelings of guilt and resentment towards the patient, which can further impact the caregiving relationship.

Lack of Training and Support: Many caregivers may not have the necessary training or support to care for an Alzheimer's patient or loved one. They may not know how to handle the behavioral changes or understand the disease's progression. This lack of knowledge can lead to feelings of frustration and helplessness.

Grief and Loss: Alzheimer's disease is a progressive disease, and caregivers may experience grief and loss as they watch their loved one's cognitive abilities decline and they "lose" the parent, sibling or friend they knew. This can be incredibly taxing to cope with and can further impact the caregiver's own mental health.

Complex Care Needs: As Alzheimer's disease progresses, the patient's care needs become more complex. The caregiver may need to assist with activities of daily living, such as bathing,dressing and personal hygiene; activities that both a patient and caregiver may find uncomfortable because of the intimacy required or perceived gender roles They may also need to manage medications and monitor the patient's health. This can be incredibly challenging, especially for caregivers who are not trained in healthcare.

Lack of Control: Alzheimer's disease can be unpredictable, and caregivers may feel like they have lost control over their lives. They may not know what to expect from day to day, and this uncertainty can be unsettling. This lack of control can lead to feelings of anxiety and depression.

Stigma: There is still a stigma surrounding Alzheimer's disease, and caregivers may feel ashamed or embarrassed to talk about their caregiving role. This can further isolate them from their support network and lead to feelings of loneliness and depression.

It is important for caregivers to prioritize their own self-care and seek out resources and support to help navigate this difficult role. It is also important to increase awareness and reduce the stigma surrounding Alzheimer's disease to support both patients and caregivers.

5.2 Legal and Financial Considerations

Planning for the legal and financial future is critical for those with Alzheimer's disease and their families and caregivers. The costs associated with Alzheimer's disease including medical bills, costs of prescriptions, nursing care, and long-term care can add up and quickly drain personal savings. It's important to have your legal matters such as a will and powers of attorney settled before the disease progresses. If you or a loved one has been diagnosed with Alzheimer's, ideally you've planned certain legal and financial matters in advance, such as:

- Completing a will
- Having a power of attorney
- Arranging for long-term care

If those and other legal and financial protections are not in place, you and your family member should move quickly to get certain protections in order.

Now how do you manage your legal and financial matters when set:

Take Action While You Can: The legal competency rule means that a person must be considered competent in the eyes of the law to make decisions regarding legal and financial matters, such as preparing one's will.

People in the early stages of Alzheimer's may be quite competent (that is, still able to understand and make decisions about their own legal or financial affairs). A court does not automatically assume that an Alzheimer's patient is legally incompetent. However, a competent patient with a recent Alzheimer's diagnosis must not delay putting legal and financial protections in place before the disease progresses further.

If someone is in the more advanced stages of the disease, a court may determine that he or she is legally incompetent. If so, and there is agreement, the person's family or friends may be able to manage affairs. But the court may appoint a surrogate to legally act on behalf of the person with Alzheimer's.

Create Durable Powers of Attorney: The competent individual should establish two types of durable power of attorney:

- Durable power of attorney for health care: Sometimes known as a living will, this type of power of attorney allows the patient to appoint a trusted person to make health care decisions for the patient when he or she can no longer do so. These decisions cover both minor and major medical issues, including life support and end-of-life care, and may contain a "Do Not Resuscitate" order. The patient's physician should have a copy of this document.

- Durable power of attorney for finances: This type enables a person to authorize a family member, friend or professional to act as an agent or proxy once he or she becomes incapacitated. This individual makes financial decisions on behalf of the Alzheimer's patient in areas like banking, investments, tax, and retirement. If these powers of attorney were not named before the individual became incapacitated, a court may have to establish a conservator for financial matters. (The conservator does not make health decisions.) This process can be very slow and expensive. That's one of many reasons that it's best to establish durable powers of attorney as soon as possible while the Alzheimer's patient is capable of handling his or her affairs.

People with Alzheimer's may want to establish a living trust, which must be done while the person is still alive. The person designates someone to serve as the trustee, who manages trust assets and then ensures their proper distribution after the patient's death.

Have a Will in Place: A will details how an individual's assets and estate will be divided upon his or her death. A person must be of sound mind to make a will, so it's best to have a will in place before a diagnosis of Alzheimer's.

For the newly diagnosed Alzheimer's patient, determine whether a will has been completed and is up to date. If there is no will but the patient is still legally competent, he or she will need to move quickly to have one completed.

If a person dies with no will, then the state will determine how assets should be distributed—typically to spouses, children, or other family members.

Get Good Legal Advice: A lawyer can help interpret state laws, draft and update necessary documents, and ensure that the wishes of the patient are followed.

You may have a trusted family lawyer to advise you. Another option is an attorney who specializes in elder law. This is an expert on the legal issues of aging, including:

- Long-term care

- Taxes
- Estate planning
- Medicare
- Medicaid

5.3 Balancing Caregiving with Personal Life

It's a constant juggle to take care of a loved one with Alzheimer's and also maintain a full-time job. The stress and exhaustion of caregiving can impact the caregiver's personal and professional life. As a caregiver, it is important to remember that your self-care is equally important as the care you provide your loved ones. In this subchapter, we will outline some strategies and tools to help you navigate work-life balance while caring for someone with Alzheimer's.

Schedule and Prioritize: Managing time is crucial when it comes to balancing caregiving and work, and the need to plan, set goals and prioritize daily tasks is critical to creating this balance. Start by creating a schedule that allows for flexibility, including time slots for caregiving tasks and time for work-related activities. Prioritize your most important tasks for each day and try to get them done first.

Seek Support: Caregiving can be a solitary experience, and it's easy to feel isolated and overwhelmed. It's essential to have support from others who can help share the burden. Contact friends and family members who can lend you a hand or provide emotional support. Look for local caregiver support groups where you can meet other caregivers dealing with similar challenges. Don't forget to visit your Uprise Health EAP care navigator for assistance in connecting with groups locally.

Take Care of Your Health: It's easy to put your own physical and emotional wellness on the back burner when caring for a loved one. But taking care of yourself is vital for maintaining your energy and resilience. Try to eat healthily, stay hydrated, and get enough rest. Exercise regularly, even if it's just a few minutes a day, as it can help release stress and tension.

Set Realistic Expectations: It's easy to become overwhelmed when caregiving, and being honest about what you can realistically handle is important. Avoid overcommitting and become comfortable with saying no when necessary. Letting go of perfectionism and embracing the imperfections of caregiving can reduce anxiety and stress levels.

Consider Professional Help: There are instances when you may need professional help to manage the care of your loved one with Alzheimer's. A professional caregiver can be hired a few hours a day, or more if necessary, so you can focus on work or attend to your needs. Consider utilizing respite care for a short break, which can be a refreshing and beneficial escape from your caregiving responsibilities.

It's easy to feel alone and overstressed while balancing caregiving and work. Remember, you are not alone in this situation. Setting realistic expectations for yourself, getting the help you need, and communicating your needs to your employer, co-workers, and family members is essential. Above all else, take care of your health and well-being. With a bit of planning, support from others, and a commitment to self-care, you can successfully navigate work-life balance while caring for someone with Alzheimer's.

Chapter 6: Effective Communication

6.1 Communicating with a Loved One with Alzheimer's

Communicating with a loved one with Alzheimer's disease requires patience and understanding. Each day may bring new challenges for caregivers and caring for your loved one can be difficult and overwhelming at times. But these tips can help both you and your loved one understand and communicate more effectively with each other.

Listen respectfully and compassionately: Seeing a loved one struggle with paranoia, agitation, or repetitive actions (all signs of Alzheimer's disease) can be upsetting. But, remember, what they're experiencing is very real to them. Do not argue, disagree, or take it personally. Listen to their struggles and distract them or redirect their focus on other activities if needed. Give your loved one plenty of time to respond to questions or gather their thoughts before speaking. Take the time to listen patiently and allow them to express their thoughts, feelings, and needs to you in their own way.

Do Not Talk About Your Loved One Like They're Not in the Room: Don't exclude them from conversations about their disease or treatment, and don't make assumptions about their ability to communicate because of their diagnosis. Alzheimer's disease affect everyone differently. Speak directly to them and ask what they are comfortable doing or what they feel they may need help with. As their disease progresses, this may not be an option, but in the earlier stages of memory loss, your loved one may still be able to participate in meaningful conversations about their quality of life.

Keep it Simple: Ask one question or give one direction at a time, especially if your loved one does not remember how to perform daily tasks. Speak slowly and clearly. Ask yes or no questions rather than open-ended ones (i.e., Do you want a drink of water? vs. What drink would you like?). Offer clear, simple, step-by-step instructions for tasks as needed. Lengthy requests may be overwhelming to them.

Stay Positive: Unfortunately, Alzheimer's has its ups and downs. There will be good days, and there will be bad days. Do not use offensive language or negative statements, even if your loved one has done so or you feel frustrated. Avoid arguing, be patient, and offer reassurance. Avoid criticizing or correcting. Instead, listen and try to find meaning in what they say. It's okay to repeat your loved one's words back to you for clarification. It's also okay to laugh. Sometimes humor can lighten the mood and make tough conversations easier.

Eliminate Distractions: Engage your loved one in one-on-one conversations in a quiet space. As their disease progresses, your loved one may struggle to pay attention or communicate with distractions like the TV, cell phones, or too many people are around. Set them up for success when communicating by lessening these disruptions.

Don't Pull Away or Avoid Them: Your honesty, love, and support are important to your loved one. It's okay if you don't always know what to say. Sometimes just being present and listening is enough. Maintain eye contact, it's a simple way to show your loved one that you care about them and what they are saying.

Encourage Nonverbal Communication: Struggling to understand what your loved one is trying to tell you? Ask them to point to objects or gesture. Use your senses—touch, sight, sounds, smells, and tastes—as communication, if able. You may need to rely on facial expressions or vocal sounds to determine your loved one's needs. Pay attention to these and respond accordingly.

Allow Them to Feel Safe and Secure: Especially in later stages of Alzheimer's disease, approach your loved one from the front and identify yourself. If they do not immediately recognize you, they may feel frightened or angry. If your loved one becomes upset or angry, try changing the subject or distracting and redirecting their energy. For example, if you ask them to eat a snack and they become angry, acknowledge how they feel and suggest going for a walk or listening to music instead. Maintain structure and security by keeping the same routines, too.

Remember the Good Times: Sharing good memories is a relaxing way to connect with your loved one. Many people with Alzheimer's disease struggle with short-term memory, but they can recall details from their lives nearly 50 years ago. Connect with your loved one over old photographs or ask about people, places, and activities from years ago.

Seek Outside Help, You Don't Have to do It Alone: As Alzheimer's disease progress, it's normal to feel a significant loss. Lean on other caregivers and family members for support. Attend a support group in your area, schedule weekly check-ins with all family members to discuss caregiving responsibilities and know when it's time to ask for additional help. Talk to your loved one's doctor about significant behavioral changes to understand the triggers of these behaviors.

6.2 Dealing with Challenging Behaviors

The most important thing that caregivers need to remember is that challenging behaviors may not be entirely avoidable. It's also not the fault of the person with Alzheimer's. These behaviors are sometimes a common product of the disease. And, there is specialized support a caregiver can use to help keep a challenging behavior from escalating.

While there is no guaranteed approach that will work with every person or situation, there are some methods that can help caregivers manage trying times:

Staying Calm: It's not uncommon for caregivers to feel attacked or helpless when they are caring for someone exhibiting difficult behaviors. Remembering that it isn't personal and that it's a symptom of the disease, can help caregivers manage their emotions and avoid contributing to tense or difficult situations. Arguing or reasoning can often escalate an outburst, so it's necessary for caregivers to stay calm and supportive.

Keeping a Schedule: People that suffer from Alzheimer's disease often find it reassuring to have a set schedule for meals, activities and daily tasks. Creating a schedule, and sticking to it as much as possible, can help prevent anxiety, confusion and anger.

Exercise: Exercise, with approval from a physician, is a great stress reliever for both seniors and caregivers. And, participating in activities together helps foster important emotional connections.

Participating in Activities: Whether it's an enjoyable hobby, household chore or physician-approved exercise, participating in joyful activities has shown to help manage challenging behaviors. These can be pre-scheduled or introduced when difficult behaviors are recognized. For example, caregivers can ask for help folding laundry to ease anxiety or can play music or sing to calm someone feeling confused, angry or depressed.

Mindful Communication: Caregivers shouldn't underestimate the power of communication. Caregivers can use soothing tones, speak in a friendly way and make eye contact to convey normalcy, understanding and compassion. This can help seniors experiencing anxiety or frustration to calm themselves.

Chapter 7: Creating a Safe and Supportive Environment

7.1 Home Safety Tips

If safety measures are in place, an individual living with Alzheimer's can live in the comfort of his or her own home or a caregiver's residence. As the disease progresses, the person's abilities will change. But with some creativity and flexibility, the home can be adapted to support these changes. Here are home safety tips you may want to consider in creating a safe environment:

Evaluate Your Environment: A person living with Alzheimer's may be more prone to safety hazards in certain areas of the home or outdoors. Monitor garages, work rooms, basements and outside areas, where there are more likely to be tools, chemicals, cleaning supplies and other potentially hazardous items.

Avoid Safety Hazards in the Kitchen: Use appliances that have an automatic shut-off feature. Prevent unsafe stove usage by applying stove knob covers, removing knobs or turning off the gas when the stove is not in use. Disconnect the garbage disposal. Discard toxic plants and decorative fruits that may be mistaken for real food. Remove vitamins, prescription drugs, sugar substitutes and seasonings from the kitchen table and counters.

Be Prepared for Emergencies: Keep a list of emergency phone numbers and addresses for local police and fire departments, hospitals and poison control helplines.

Make Sure Safety Devices are in Working Order: Make sure carbon monoxide and smoke detectors and fire extinguishers are available and inspected regularly. Replace batteries twice a year during daylight saving time.

Install Locks Out of Sight: Place a latch or deadbolt either above or below eye level on all doors. Remove locks on interior doors to prevent the person living with Alzheimer's from locking themselves in. Keep an extra set of keys hidden near the door for easy access.

Keep Walkways and Rooms Well-Lit: Changes in levels of light can be disorienting. Create an even level by adding extra lights in entries, outside landings, and areas between rooms, stairways and bathrooms. Use night lights in hallways, bedrooms and bathrooms.

Consider Removing Guns and Other Weapons from the Home or Storing Them in a Locked Cabinet: If someone in the home is living with Alzheimer's or another dementia, firearms can pose a significant risk for everyone. For example, as the disease progresses, the person may not recognize someone he or she has known for years and view him or her as an intruder. With a gun accessible, the result could be disastrous.

Place Medications in a Locked Drawer or Cabinet: To help ensure that medications are taken safely, use a pill box organizer or keep a daily list and check off each medication as it is taken.

Remove Tripping Hazards: Remove throw rugs, extension cords and excessive clutter.

Watch the Temperature of Water and Food: It may be difficult for the person living with Alzheimer's to tell the difference between hot and cold. Consider installing an automatic thermometer for water temperature.

Assess Bedroom Safety: Closely monitor the use of an electric blanket, heater or heating pad to prevent burns or other injuries. Provide seating near the bed to help with dressing. Ensure closet shelves are at an accessible height so that items are easy to reach, which may prevent the person from climbing shelves or objects falling from overhead.

Secure Large Furniture: Check that book shelves, cabinets or large TVs are secured to prevent tipping. Ensure chairs have armrests to provide support when going from a sitting to standing position.

Avoid Injury in the Bathroom: Install grab bars for the shower, tub and toilet to provide additional support: Apply textured stickers to slippery surfaces to prevent falls. Consider installing a walk-in shower.

Support the Person's Needs: Try not to create a home that feels too restrictive. The home should encourage independence and social interaction. Clear areas for activities.

7.2 Daily Routine and Structure

Daily routines can be helpful for both you the caregiver and the person living with Alzheimer's. A planned day allows you to spend less time trying to figure out what to do, and more time on activities that provide meaning and enjoyment.

First, you need to organize your day, remember to make time for yourself, or include the person living with Alzheimer's in activities that you enjoy for example, taking a daily walk. A person with Alzheimer's will eventually need a caregiver's assistance to organize the day. Structured and pleasant activities can often reduce agitation and improve mood. Planning activities for a person with Alzheimer's works best when you continually explore, experiment and adjust.

Before making a plan, consider:

- The person's likes, dislikes, strengths, abilities and interests
- How the person used to structure his or her day
- What times of day the person functions best
- Ample time for meals, bathing and dressing
- Regular times for waking up and going to bed (especially helpful if the person with dementia experiences sleep issues or sundowning)
- Make sure to allow for flexibility within your daily routine for spontaneous activities.

As Alzheimer's disease progresses, the abilities of a person with the disease will change. With creativity, flexibility and problem solving, you'll be able to adapt your daily routine to support these changes.

Second, you need to write a plan when thinking about organizing the day, consider:

- Which activities work best? Which don't? Why? (Keep in mind that the success of an activity can vary from day-to-day.)
- Are there times when there is too much going on or too little to do?
- Were spontaneous activities enjoyable or did they create anxiety and confusion?

Don't be concerned about filling every minute with an activity. The person with Alzheimer's needs a balance of activity and rest, and may need more frequent breaks and varied tasks. In general, if the person seems bored, distracted or irritable, it may be time to introduce another activity or to take time out for rest. The type of activity and how well it's completed are not as important as the joy and sense of accomplishment the person gets from doing it.

7.3 Managing Medications and Appointments

In the early stages of Alzheimer's, the person may need help remembering to take medications. As a caregiver, you may find it helpful to:

Use a Pill Box Organizer: Using a pill box or keeping a daily list or calendar can help ensure medication is taken as prescribed.

Develop a Routine for Giving the Medication: Ask the pharmacist how medications should be taken at a certain time of the day or with or without food. Then create a daily routine, such as taking medications with meals or before bed

As the disease progresses, you'll need to provide a greater level of care. In addition to using a pill box organizer and keeping a daily routine, try these tips:

Use Simple Language and Clear Instructions: For example, say "Here's the pill for your high blood pressure. Put it in your mouth and drink some water." If the person refuses to take the medication, stop and try again later.

If Swallowing is a Problem, Ask if the Medication is Available in Another Form: Talk to the doctor who prescribed the medication or the pharmacist to find out if a liquid version is available or if it is safe to crush the medication and mix it with food. Be aware that no pill or tablet should be crushed without first consulting your physician or pharmacist, since it can cause some medications to be ineffective or unsafe.

Make Changes for Safety: Be sure to place medications in a locked drawer or cabinet to avoid accidental overdose, and throw out medications that are no longer being used or that have expired.

Have Emergency Numbers Easily Accessible: Keep the number of your local poison control center or emergency room handy. If you suspect a medication overdose, call poison control or 911 before taking any action.

Chapter 8: Self-Care for Caregivers

8.1 Recognizing Burnout and Compassion Fatigue

Caregiver burnout is a state of physical, emotional and mental exhaustion that can happen when you dedicate time and energy to manage the health and safety of someone else. Caregivers who experience burnout may feel tired, stressed, withdrawn, anxious and depressed. Caregiver burnout can impact a person in various ways, including physically, psychologically, financially and socially.

Burnout feels like a candle that ran out of a wick, it doesn't have what it needs to continue to provide light. It can occur when you don't get the help you need personally, as you devote all of your time and energy to helping someone else. It can also happen when you try to do more than you're able to, emotionally, physically or financially.

Your health and well-being matter just as much as the person you're caring for. It's important to know the signs and symptoms of caregiver burnout so you can get the help you need when you need it most.

Recognizing caregiver burnout is similar to that of a person who is stressed and depressed. The following are the symptoms to enable you recognize:

- Emotional and physical exhaustion.
- Withdrawal from friends, family and other loved ones.

- Loss of interest in activities previously enjoyed.
- Feeling hopeless and helpless.
- Changes in appetite and/or weight.
- Changes in sleep patterns.
- Unable to concentrate.
- Getting sick more often.
- Irritability, frustration or anger toward others.

If at any time you feel overwhelmed, you need someone to talk to or you're thinking about hurting yourself or suicide, call or text 988 to reach the Suicide and Crisis Lifeline (U.S.). Someone is available to help you 24/7. If your burnout causes resentment toward the person you're caring for or you feel like you may be hurting that person, reach out for help immediately. You could contact a friend or family member, a healthcare provider, a social worker or a mental health professional.

Compassion fatigue is considered a secondary stress disorder resulting from a care recipient's high level of emotional stress. Studies have shown that correctional workers, counselors, nurses and some social workers have a high risk of the condition because of their work environments. Caregiver burnout is a common phenomenon amongst caregivers, but compassion fatigue is not so widely known.

8.2 Strategies for Self-Care

Being an Alzheimer's caregiver can be a challenging and emotionally draining role. It can be difficult to balance your own needs with those of your loved one, and it's not uncommon for caregivers to experience burnout and stress.

That's why incorporating self-care into your daily routine is so important. Taking care of yourself can help you better care for your loved one and improve your overall well-being.

Asking for Help: Taking care of yourself when caring for someone with Alzheimer's is an essential part of being a caregiver. As a caregiver, it's important to identify your support network and be honest about what you need and how you feel. It can be challenging to recognize and understand the support that exists around you, especially when caring for a loved one with Alzheimer's can be overwhelming and emotionally taxing. However, self-care is essential to maintain both physical and mental health. Finding individuals or organizations that can help you manage tasks or offer emotional support can provide much-needed relief.

Join a Caregiver's Support Group: As a caregiver for someone with Alzheimer's, it's important to connect with local support groups. These groups can provide a safe space for individuals to share their experiences and find comfort in others who understand the struggles of caring for someone with Alzheimer's. In-person groups offer the opportunity for face-to-face interaction and provide a sense of community. Online groups can offer convenience, anonymity, and access to a wider range of people. Regardless of the type of support group, participating in these groups can help improve your overall well-being.

Taking Care of Yourself: When you are caring for someone with Alzheimer's, it can be easy to put their needs before your own. However, it's essential to prioritize self-care to ensure you remain healthy and well-rested. It's important to make time for activities that bring you joy, such as exercise, reading, or spending time with friends and family. You should also make sure you are getting enough sleep and eating a balanced diet to support your physical health. Neglecting your own well-being can have serious consequences, including burnout and increased stress levels. By taking care of yourself, you can better care for your loved one with Alzheimer's and maintain your own quality of life. Remember that self-care is not selfish, but rather a crucial aspect of being a responsible caregiver.

8.3 Respite Care and Seeking Help

Everyone needs a break. Respite care provides caregivers a temporary rest from caregiving, while the person living with Alzheimer's continues to receive care in a safe environment. Using respite services can support and strengthen your ability to be a caregiver.

Respite care can provide:

- A chance to spend time with other friends and family, or to just relax
- Time to take care of errands such as shopping, exercising, getting a haircut or going to the doctor
- Comfort and peace of mind knowing that the person with Alzheimer's is spending time with another caring individual

Respite care services can give the person with Alzheimer an opportunity to:

- Interact with others having similar experiences

- Spend time in a safe, supportive environment
- Participate in activities designed to match personal abilities and needs

PART III: Strategies and Resources

Chapter 9: Lifestyle and Alzheimer's

9.1 Nutrition and Diet

Regular, nutritious meals may become a challenge for people living in the middle and late stages of Alzheimer's. They may become overwhelmed with too many food choices, forget to eat or think they have already eaten. Proper nutrition is important to keep the body strong and healthy. For a person with Alzheimer's, poor nutrition may increase behavioral symptoms and cause weight loss.

The basic nutrition tips below can help boost the health of the Alzheimer's patient and your health as a caregiver, too.

Provide a Balanced Diet With a Variety of Foods: Offer vegetables, fruits, whole grains, low-fat dairy products and lean protein foods.

Limit Foods with High Saturated Fat and Cholesterol: Some fat is essential for health but not all fats are equal. Go light on fats that are bad for heart health, such as butter, solid shortening, lard and fatty cuts of meat.

Cut Down on Refined Sugars: Often found in processed foods, refined sugars contain calories but lack vitamins, minerals and fiber. You can tame a sweet tooth with healthier options like fruit or juice-sweetened baked goods. But note that in the later-stages of Alzheimer's, if appetite loss is a problem, adding sugar to foods may encourage eating.

Limit Foods With High Sodium and Use Less Salt: Most people in the United States consume too much sodium, which affects blood pressure. As an alternative, use spices or herbs to season food.

As the disease progresses, loss of appetite and weight loss may become concerns. In such cases, the doctor may suggest supplements between meals to add calories. Staying hydrated may also be a problem. Encourage fluid intake by offering small cups of water or other liquids throughout the day or foods with high water content such as fruit, soups, milkshakes and smoothies.

9.2 Exercise and Physical Activity

Engaging in regular exercise and physical activity is a vital component of Alzheimer's care, even in the middle stages of the disease. Physical activity can help maintain and enhance the patient's overall wellbeing, cognitive function, and quality of life. Here's a detailed perspective on the importance of exercise and physical activity in Alzheimer's care:

Cognitive Benefits: Exercise has been shown to have a positive impact on cognitive function, even in individuals with Alzheimer's disease. Physical activity can help preserve memory, attention, and problem-solving skills. While it may not reverse the course of the disease, it can slow down cognitive decline and provide a sense of accomplishment and satisfaction for patients.

Improved Physical Health: Regular exercise contributes to better physical health, promoting cardiovascular health, reducing the risk of chronic conditions such as heart disease and diabetes, and maintaining muscle strength and joint flexibility. This can enhance the patient's ability to perform daily activities and reduce the risk of complications.

Mood and Emotional Wellbeing: Physical activity has a direct impact on mood and emotional wellbeing. Engaging in exercise releases endorphins, which can alleviate symptoms of depression, anxiety, and stress that often accompany Alzheimer's. Exercise can also help improve sleep patterns, reducing sleep disturbances common in Alzheimer's patients.

Enhanced Quality of Life: Staying active contributes to an improved quality of life. It can foster a sense of accomplishment and independence, allowing patients to take charge of their health and maintain a higher level of autonomy for longer. Additionally, physical activity can enhance social interactions, fostering a sense of belonging and emotional support.

Caregiver Support: Engaging in physical activity can provide a sense of structure and routine for patients, which can make caregiving more manageable. Caregivers often find that exercise programs help reduce challenging behaviors, enhance the patient's mood, and provide meaningful activities to share.

Tailored Exercise Programs: The middle stages of Alzheimer's require tailored exercise programs that consider the patient's abilities and limitations. Simple activities such as walking, chair exercises, or gentle yoga can be adapted to meet the individual's needs. Supervision and support from caregivers or healthcare professionals may be necessary to ensure safety.

Consistency and Routine: Establishing a regular exercise routine is important. Consistency can help patients become familiar with the activity, making it less intimidating. It also creates a sense of predictability, which can reduce anxiety and frustration.

Safety Precautions: Safety is a top priority when implementing exercise programs for Alzheimer's patients. Exercises should be done in a safe environment, free of obstacles or hazards. Patients may require assistance or supervision, especially if balance or mobility is compromised.

Adjusting as the Disease Progresses: Alzheimer's is a progressive disease, and the patient's abilities may change over time. It's crucial to adjust exercise routines and activities accordingly. The emphasis should always be on safe and enjoyable physical activity that supports the patient's overall health and wellbeing.

Incorporating exercise and physical activity into Alzheimer's care during the middle stages of the disease can be a transformative strategy. It not only contributes to cognitive and physical health but also fosters emotional wellbeing and a higher quality of life. Whether engaging in simple stretching exercises, walking, or more structured programs, the goal is to maintain physical and mental vitality while providing a sense of achievement and fulfillment for the patient. It is important to consult with healthcare professionals and caregivers to develop a personalized exercise plan tailored to the patient's specific needs and abilities.

9.3 Cognitive Stimulation

Cognitive stimulation is a fundamental aspect of Alzheimer's care, especially during the middle stages of the disease. While Alzheimer's presents cognitive challenges, engaging in activities that stimulate the mind can help maintain cognitive function, slow down cognitive decline, and improve the patient's overall quality of life. Here's a detailed perspective on the importance of cognitive stimulation in Alzheimer's care:

Cognitive Preservation: The middle stages of Alzheimer's often involve a significant decline in cognitive function, particularly memory, problem-solving, and language abilities. Engaging in cognitive stimulation activities can help preserve these functions to some extent. These activities challenge the brain, encouraging it to remain active and maintain its cognitive capabilities.

Enhanced Memory: Memory-related activities, such as puzzles or memory games, can assist in enhancing memory retention. While Alzheimer's may impair short-term memory, it's common for patients to retain long-term memories. Engaging in reminiscence activities and discussing past experiences can be emotionally rewarding and support the preservation of memories.

Problem-Solving and Critical Thinking: Cognitive stimulation activities often involve problem-solving and critical thinking exercises. Engaging in such activities can improve the patient's ability to think logically, make decisions, and navigate daily life. These exercises can also enhance a sense of independence and self-esteem.

Communication Skills: Activities that promote conversation, storytelling, and interaction with others can support the patient's communication skills. Engaging in conversations and discussions, even if memory is compromised, can provide opportunities for social engagement and emotional connections.

Emotional Wellbeing: Cognitive stimulation can have a positive impact on emotional wellbeing. It can reduce feelings of frustration, boredom, and isolation often experienced by Alzheimer's patients. Engaging in mentally stimulating activities provides a sense of accomplishment and a boost in self-esteem.

Personalized Approach: Cognitive stimulation activities should be tailored to the individual's abilities and interests. Some patients may enjoy word games, while others might prefer art, music, or reading. A personalized approach ensures the patient finds the activities engaging and enjoyable.

Regular Routine: Consistency in cognitive stimulation activities is crucial. A regular routine can provide structure and predictability, reducing anxiety and agitation. Patients often benefit from knowing what to expect, especially during the middle stages of Alzheimer's when confusion and disorientation can be prevalent.

Caregiver Involvement:Caregivers play a crucial role in facilitating cognitive stimulation activities. They can provide guidance, structure, and emotional support during these activities. Caregivers can also monitor the patient's responses to tailor activities to their changing needs.

Adapting to Changing Abilities: Alzheimer's is a progressive disease, and the patient's cognitive abilities may change over time. It's essential to adapt cognitive stimulation activities to match the patient's current capabilities. Flexibility in the approach is key to providing meaningful engagement.

Cognitive stimulation is not only about preserving cognitive function but also about fostering a sense of accomplishment, purpose, and social connection for Alzheimer's patients. It provides a way for them to engage actively in their own care, stimulating the mind and improving overall wellbeing. By working closely with healthcare professionals and caregivers to tailor cognitive stimulation activities to the patient's needs and preferences, individuals with Alzheimer's can continue to lead fulfilling and meaningful lives, even in the face of cognitive challenges.

Chapter 10: Promising Therapies and Research

10.1 Current Treatment Options

Several prescription drugs are approved by the U.S. Food and Drug Administration (FDA) for Alzheimer's disease to help either manage the symptoms or to treat the disease. Most FDA-approved drugs work best for people in the early or middle stages of Alzheimer's. There are currently no known interventions that will cure Alzheimer's.

Medications for Mild to Moderate Alzheimer's Disease

Treating the symptoms of Alzheimer's can help provide people with comfort, dignity, and independence for a longer period of time and also assist their caregivers. Galantamine, rivastigmine, and donepezil are cholinesterase inhibitors that are prescribed for mild to moderate Alzheimer's symptoms. These drugs may help reduce or control some cognitive and behavioral symptoms.

Cholinesterase inhibitors prevent the breakdown of acetylcholine, a brain chemical believed to be important for memory and thinking. As Alzheimer's progresses, the brain produces less acetylcholine and, over time, these medicines lose their effectiveness. Because cholinesterase inhibitors work in a similar way, switching from one to another may not produce significantly different results but a person living with Alzheimer's may respond better to one drug versus another.

Lecanemab is an FDA-approved immunotherapy to treat early Alzheimer's. It targets the protein beta-amyloid to help reduce amyloid plaques, one of the hallmark brain changes in Alzheimer's. Clinical studies to determine the effectiveness of lecanemab were conducted only in people with early-stage Alzheimer's, or mild cognitive impairment due to the disease. Study results showed lecanemab slowed the rate of cognitive decline among study participants over the course of 18 months and reduced the levels of amyloid in the brain. Currently, insurance may only cover this medication in specific situations.

The FDA granted accelerated approval for aducanumab, which is also an immunotherapy used to treat early Alzheimer's. To gain full FDA approval, the drug company must conduct additional studies on the clinical benefits of the drug. Currently, insurance may only cover this medication in specific situations.

Before prescribing these medications, doctors may order PET scans or an analysis of cerebrospinal fluid to evaluate whether amyloid deposits are present in the brain. There are possible side effects to taking these medications, including brain swelling or bleeding. In rare instances, these side effects may be serious and life-threatening. Due to this potential risk, monitoring with routine MRIs is required.

Several other medications to treat Alzheimer's are being tested in people with mild cognitive impairment or early Alzheimer's.

Medications for Moderate to Severe Alzheimer's Disease

A medication known as memantine, an N-methyl-D-aspartate (NMDA) antagonist, can be prescribed for moderate to severe Alzheimer's. This drug is prescribed to decrease symptoms, which could enable some people to maintain certain daily functions a little longer than they would without the medication. For example, memantine may help a person in the later stages of the disease maintain their ability to use the bathroom independently for several more months, a benefit for both people with Alzheimer's and their caregivers.

Memantine is believed to work by regulating glutamate, an important brain chemical. When produced in excessive amounts, glutamate may lead to brain cell death. Because NMDA antagonists work differently from cholinesterase inhibitors, the two types of drugs can be prescribed in combination.

The FDA has also approved donepezil, the rivastigmine patch, and a combination medication of memantine and donepezil for moderate to severe Alzheimer's.

Brexpiprazole is an atypical antipsychotic that has been approved to treat agitation associated with Alzheimer's. See below for more information on managing behavioral symptoms and antipsychotics.

10.2 Emerging Therapies and Clinical Trials

Emerging therapies and clinical trials hold the promise of revolutionizing the way we approach Alzheimer's care. These innovative approaches are at the forefront of the battle against the disease, and while not all are proven, they offer hope for better treatment and management:

Immunotherapies: Immunotherapies are a class of treatments that aim to harness the body's immune system to target and clear the abnormal protein deposits in the brain, such as beta-amyloid. Monoclonal antibodies like Aducanumab and Lecanemab are being studied in clinical trials to determine their effectiveness in removing amyloid plaques and potentially slowing cognitive decline.

Anti-Tau Therapies: Emerging therapies targeting tau protein abnormalities are another area of active research. Abnormal tau tangles are strongly associated with Alzheimer's progression. Drugs like LMTM (LMTX) and

ALZ-801 are being evaluated to reduce tau pathology.

Small Molecule Therapies: Small molecules are compounds designed to influence cellular processes implicated in Alzheimer's. Some drugs target enzymes and receptors involved in the disease, with the goal of modifying its course. One example is TRx0237 (LMTX), which is undergoing clinical trials.

Gene Therapies: Gene therapies aim to modify or replace genes associated with Alzheimer's to influence disease progression. Clinical trials are exploring the use of gene therapies to modify the expression of specific genes linked to the disease.

Lifestyle Interventions: Lifestyle interventions encompass a holistic approach to Alzheimer's care. Exercise, diet, cognitive engagement, and sleep management are all integral components. These interventions aim to address multiple factors influencing Alzheimer's progression and overall health.

Disease-Modifying Therapies: A major focus of emerging therapies is to develop treatments that can modify the course of the disease by addressing its underlying causes. These therapies hold the potential to slow or halt cognitive decline rather than just managing symptoms.

Biomarker-Driven Treatment: Emerging therapies often take a personalized approach by utilizing biomarkers and genetic information. This allows for the tailoring of treatments to the specific characteristics of each patient's disease, enabling more precise and effective care.

Combination Therapies: Some clinical trials are exploring the effectiveness of combining multiple treatments or interventions to target different aspects of Alzheimer's disease simultaneously. These combination approaches aim to provide a more comprehensive and effective treatment strategy.

Early Intervention: Early detection and intervention are becoming increasingly important. By identifying Alzheimer's in its earliest stages, emerging therapies can be administered when they are most likely to be effective in modifying the disease's course.

Ethical Considerations: As emerging therapies advance, ethical concerns related to consent, data privacy, and equitable access come to the forefront. These considerations are crucial to ensure that patients are well-informed, involved in the decision-making process, and treated with respect and fairness.

Ongoing Research: It's important to recognize that not all emerging therapies will prove effective, and the path to regulatory approval is rigorous. Ongoing research, clinical trials, and regulatory processes are integral to evaluating the safety and efficacy of these treatments.

Emerging therapies and clinical trials offer a ray of hope in the ongoing battle against Alzheimer's disease. They represent the cutting edge of research and development, with the potential to transform the treatment landscape. Patients, caregivers, and healthcare professionals should stay informed about the latest advancements in Alzheimer's care and consider participation in clinical trials as a way to access these innovative treatments and contribute to the quest for a breakthrough in Alzheimer's management.

10.3 The Search for a Cure

Many diseases that were once fatal no longer are due to breakthroughs in medications and vaccines. HIV, smallpox and polio are just a few modern examples. Because we've successfully cured or at least learned how to properly treat these illnesses, there's hope for curing other diseases, like Alzheimer's. When it comes to Alzheimer's disease, it's impossible to predict when we will finally have a cure. Alzheimer's is difficult to understand and pin down.

Medications have been slow to develop. But as researchers gain a better understanding of the disease and what it does to the brain, we can remain hopeful that a cure is out there.

Away from this book, it would be really appreciated if you could create time to provide a review if you thought it was worthwhile, as it would motivate me. Thanks.

www.ingramcontent.com/pod-product-compliance
Lightning Source LLC
Chambersburg PA
CBHW062323290526
45794CB00005B/1867